BEST YOGA EXERCISE

SIMPLE YOGA FOR EVERYONE WITHOUT AN INSTRUCTOR

Copyright@2019

By

Dr. (PT) Jerome Coleman

Contents
Chapter 1..3
Yoga..3

Chapter 1

Yoga

In the event that you are fresh to yoga, there are sure postures that are basic for you to adapt so you can feel good in a class or rehearsing without anyone else at home.

It is not an easy one for us to discuss everything on this single book since there are more than 300 positions in the physical yoga (asana) practice, however these postures can help you in the right way.

If you manage to do these for 5-10 breaths, it will go a long way to develop you as a novice on yoga program each day.

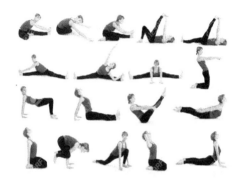

Here are my picks for the 10 most imperative yoga models for novices. Note: You don't need to have the capacity to do every one of these postures precisely as imagined — ALWAYS tune in to your body and alter if necessary.

1. Mountain Pose

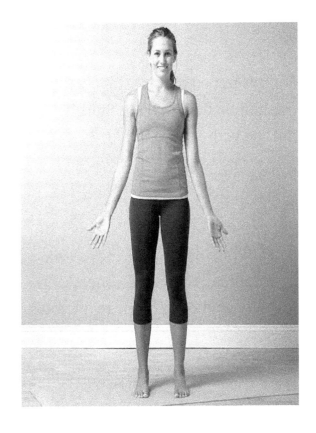

Mountain Pose is the primary stage for every single standing posture; it gives you a feeling of how to ground in to your feet and feel the earth underneath you. Mountain posture may appear to be "just standing," but there is a change taking place as you continue.

For this to be effective, follow the method on how to do it: Start by putting your feet together.

Procedures:

- Press down your toes as you spread them wide open. Draw in your quadriceps to lift your

kneecaps and lift up through the inward thighs.
- Contrast your abs and up as you raise your chest and press the highest points of the shoulders down.

- While you feel your shoulder bones coming enclose to one another and open your chest; yet keep your palms inwards towards the body.
- Assume a string drawing the head crown to the roof and inhale deeply in to the middle. Hold for 5-8 breaths.

2. Downward Facing Dog

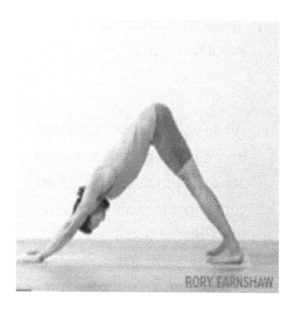

Dog Downward Dog is utilized in most yoga practices and it extends and fortifies the whole body. It is generally acceptable to say, "A down puppy daily saves you from seeing a doctor."

Step by step instructions to do it:

- Begin with every one of the fours while your wrists under your shoulders and knees under your hips.
- Tuck under your toes and lift your hips up off the floor as you step them up at back towards your heels.

- Keep your knees twisted when your hamstrings are tight, attempt and rectify your legs while holding your hips back.

- Move your hands forward to provide yourself more length in the event that you have to.

- Press immovably through your palms and turn the internal elbows towards one another.
- Free out the abs and continue drawing in your legs to keep the middle moving back towards the thighs.
- Hold for 5-8 breaths count before dropping back hands and knees to rest.

3. Board

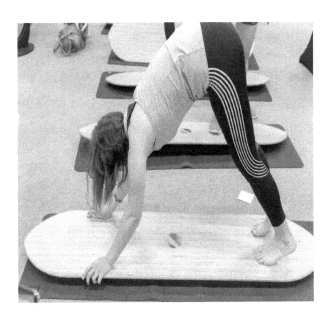

Plank shows us how to adjust staring us in the face while utilizing the whole body to help us.

It is an extraordinary method to fortify the abs, and figure out how to utilize the breath to enable us to remain in a testing present.

Step by step instructions to do it:

- From every one of the fours, tuck under your toes and lift your legs up from the tangle.

- Slide your impact points sufficiently back until the point when you believe you are one straight line of vitality from your go to your feet.

- Try to connect with the lower abs, while you draw your shoulders down and far from the ears
- Bring your ribs together and inhale profoundly for 8-10 breaths count.

4. Triangle

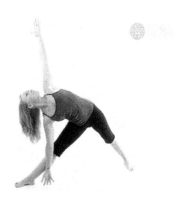

Triangle is a brilliant standing stance to extend the sides of the midriff, open up the lungs, fortify the legs and tone the whole body.

Instructions to do it:

- Start by keeping your feet while one leg's-length separated.
- Open and stretch your arms to the sides at shoulder tallness.
- Your right foot should be 90 degrees out and your left toes in around 45 degrees.

- Draw in your quadriceps and abs, while you pivot to the side over your correct leg.

- Place your correct hand down on your lower leg, shin or knee (or a square on the off chance that you have one) and lift your left arm up to the roof.

- Turn upward by looking up to the best hand and hold for 5-8 breaths.
- Lift up standing and rehash on the opposite side.

5. Tree

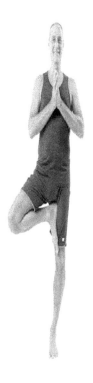

Tree Pose1Tree is a marvelous standing equalization for tenderfoots to deal with to pick up center and clearness, and figure out how to inhale while standing and keeping the body adjusted on one foot.

Step by step instructions to do it:

- Start with your feet together and raise your right foot and put it on your left inward upper thigh.
- Bring your hands in supplication and discover a

spot before you that you can hold in a watchful eye.

- Keep it up and relax for 8-10 breaths at that point change sides.
- Ensure you don't lean in to the standing leg and keep your abs connected with and shoulders loose.

6. Warrior 1

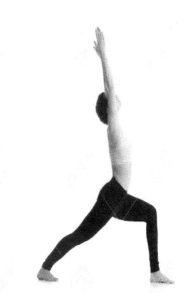

Warrior 1 postures are basically for building quality and stamina in a yoga practice.

Warrior post gives you stamina and stretches the hips and thighs in the process of building quality in the whole lower body and center.

Warrior 1 is a delicate backbend; and an incredible posture for extending open the front body while reinforcing the legs, hips, backside, center and abdominal area.

The most effective method to do it:

- For warrior one, you can make a goliath stride back with your left foot coming towards a rush, at that point turn your left impact point down and edge your left toes forward 75 degrees.

- Raise your chest and press your palms up overhead.
- Move forward and rehash on the opposite leg.

7. Warrior 2

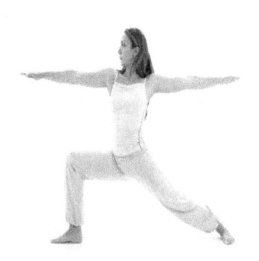

Warrior 2 pose serves to open hips and opens up the in-between thighs and crotch.

It's a decent beginning stage for some, side stances including triangle, broadened point and half-moon balance.

Step by step instructions to do it:

- Stand with your feet one leg's-length separated.
- Turn your right toes out setting 90 degrees while your left toes in 45 degrees.
- Twist your correct knee until the point that it is straightforwardly over your

correct lower leg while keeping the middle even between the hips.

- Stretch your arms to your sides and look towards your right hand.
- Keep your breaths for 8-10 before placing the right leg and turning your feet to the opposite side to rehash on left side.

8. Situated Forward Bend

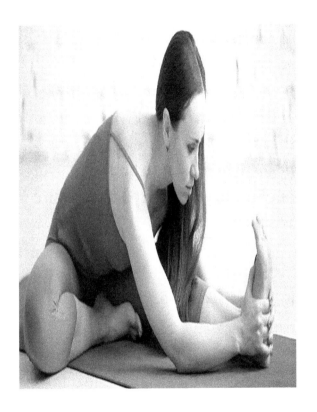

Situated Forward Fold It's imperative to consolidate a forward curve in yoga practice to extend the hamstrings, lower and upper back and sides. Situated forward curve is the ideal overlap for everybody to begin to open up the body and figure out how to inhale through awkward positions.

If during the process that you experience any sharp pain or discomfort you have to back off; yet on the off chance that you feel the strain when you crease forward and you can keep on breathing, you will gradually begin to relax up and let go.

Your knees should be kept bowed in the posture as long as the feet stay flexed and together.

The most effective method to do it:

- Start situated by placing your legs together, while your feet is firmly flexed and not turning in or out, and your hands by your hips.
- Lift your chest and start to move forward from your midsection.
- Draw in your lower abs and envision your tummy catch moving towards the highest point of your thighs.

- When you hit your most extreme, stop and relax for 8-10 breaths.
- Ensure your shoulders, head and neck are altogether discharged.

9. Scaffold Pose

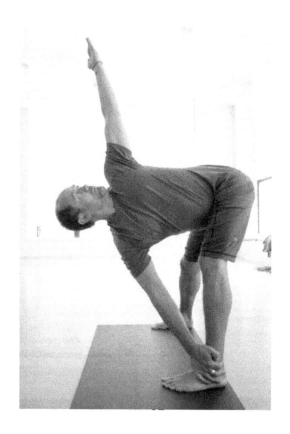

Bridge counter posture to a forward twist is a back curve. Scaffold is a decent learner's back curve that extends the front body and reinforces the back body.

Step by step instructions to do it:

- Lie down while your back is on the floor and put your feet hip width separated.
- Place your feet firmly and lift your butt up off the tangle.
- Intertwine your hands together and press the clench hands down to the floor as you open up your chest much more.

10. Child's Pose

Child's Pose Everyone needs a decent resting posture and Child's posture is a magnificent one for novices as well

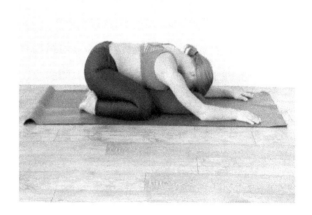

as for yoga specialists everything being equal.

It's great to gain proficiency with youngster's posture to utilize when you're exhausted in Down Dog, before bed around evening time to work out the crimps, or whenever you require a psychological break and stress/strain help.

Step by step instructions to do it:

- Start on each of the fours at that point bring your knees and feet together as you sit your butt back to your impact points and stretch your arms forward.

- Lower your chest to the floor and let your whole body discharge.
- Stay this pose for the best duration of time you can!

www.ingramcontent.com/pod-product-compliance
Lightning Source LLC
LaVergne TN
LVHW010157191224
799436LV00004B/705